Anti inflammatory Diet for Beginners

Over 100 plant-based recipes

Robert D. Paul

Contents

Chapter One

Introduction

When you first wake up in the morning, do you feel sluggish and stiff? Are you fed up with feeling exhausted and achy all of the time? You're probably looking for a long-term solution to lose weight, eat more healthfully, and regain your lost energy.

Congratulations on taking the first step toward living a healthier lifestyle by purchasing the Anti-Inflammatory Diet for Beginners book, and thank you for doing so.

In the following chapters, you will learn how to improve your quality of life, heal your immune system, lose weight, and even prevent degenerative diseases from developing. A flare-up of inflammation can send you into a downward spiral that is difficult to break free from. Pain in your muscles and joints makes you less active as a result of using these medications. A more sedentary lifestyle contributes to weight gain, which in turn increases the stress placed on your joints and causes inflammation to occur. Making dietary changes, on the other hand, can help to reduce inflammation.

The average person takes only three weeks to form a habit. Put yourself in a strong, healthy position by starting right away. In addition, there is a three-week meal plan with recipes for everything from breakfast to lunch to dinner, smoothies to dessert. With a simple change in your diet, you can significantly reduce the inflammation that contributes to fatigue, joint pain, slowed cognitive function, and a variety of autoimmune diseases, among other symptoms. You'll discover that you no longer require pain medication on a daily basis, and you won't have to starve yourself in order to accomplish this!

We appreciate you selecting this book from among the many others that are available on the subject. There has been a great deal of effort put into making this book easy to read while also including as much useful information as possible; enjoy yourself! Section 1: Introduction Irritation is defined as

It is normal for the body to experience inflammation when it is injured or infected, but it can be dangerous. It is a physiological response that signals the immune system to repair damaged cells or to fight off viruses and bacteria in the environment. Infected wounds and viruses would be lethal if there was no inflammation to signal the immune system to take action.

Although it is a good system, it is not without its faults. On occasion, inflammation manifests itself in areas of the body where it is not required. Inflammation that persists for an extended period of time is linked to diseases such as stroke and heart disease, among others.

Irritation can be classified into two types: acute and chronic inflammation. Acute inflammation occurs immediately following an injury, such as a scratch or cut, a sprained ankle, or even a sore throat. In this case, the immune system only responds to the area that has been injured.. The inflammation lasts only as long as it is necessary to repair the damage that has been caused. Blood flow would be boosted as a result of the dilation of red blood vessels. The white blood cells would multiply in the area where they were needed, assisting the body in its healing process. Redness, swelling, pain, a warm feeling, and fever are all signs of acute inflammation.

Cytokines are released by damaged tissue during acute inflammation, and they are responsible for the inflammation. When our body receives a signal from the cytokines, it sends extra white blood cells and nutrients to help the healing process along. It is a hormone-like substance called prostaglandins that causes pain and fever while also causing blood clots that aid in tissue repair. With time, the body's ability to heal itself, the inflammation diminishes until it is no longer required.

When it comes to healing the body, acute inflammation is extremely beneficial, but chronic inflammation can cause more harm than good. Chronic inflammation is generally found at low concentrations throughout the body, especially in the joints. Small increases in markers of the immune system in blood or tissue samples are frequently found to indicate the presence of this condition.

Whatever the body perceives as a threat, whether or not it is actually a threat, can trigger chronic inflammation. This inflammation still causes a response from the white blood cells; however, because there is nothing that requires their attention in order to heal, they may begin to attack healthy cells, tissues, and organs as a result of their confusion. Despite the fact that researchers are still trying to figure out how chronic inflammation works, they are aware that it increases the likelihood of developing a wide range of diseases.

Over-the-counter medications are frequently effective in treating cases of acute inflammation. The use of nonsteroidal anti-inflammatory drugs (NSAIDs) and pain relievers such as naproxen, ibuprofen, and aspirin for short-term inflammation is generally regarded as safe and effective. As a result of inhibiting the enzyme cyclooxygenase, which is responsible for the production of prostaglandins, the pain is reduced and made tolerable. If over-the-counter medications are ineffective in alleviating symptoms, prescription medications such as cortisone and steroids such as prednisone, which are known to reduce inflammation, can be used instead to help relieve symptoms. Unfortunatley, there are currently no specific drugs available for the treatment of persistent inflammation.

In the short term, there are numerous options for treating inflammation; however, all medications have side effects and may not be safe to use for an extended period of time in most cases.

It has been shown that taking nonsteroidal anti-inflammatory drugs (NSAIDs) on a regular basis for months or years increases the risk of stroke or heart attack. They also increase the risk of gastrointestinal side effects such as ulcers and bleeding. Weight gain, osteoporosis, diabetes, and muscle weakness are all possible side effects of cortisone use, according to the FDA. In addition to treating a variety of symptoms and diseases, prednisone has the side effect of suppressing the immune system, increasing the likelihood of contracting a disease. Long-term use can also increase the risk of osteoporosis, thinning skin, fluid retention, and weight gain as a result of an increased appetite caused by the medication.

Medicines can work quickly and provide pain relief for a few hours, but they also carry a number of risks and must be taken on a daily basis, usually several times a day, in order to provide long-term relief from the condition. The time to look for a safer, long-term solution to inflammation is when it becomes chronic and begins to interfere with your daily activities. As simple as altering your diet can make a significant difference. Disease Prevention (Chapter 2).

It is still difficult for researchers to grasp the specifics of inflammation and how it affects the human body. We do know that pro-inflammatory foods are associated with a higher risk of developing chronic diseases that are difficult to manage, such as type 2 diabetes and cardiovascular disease.

Your overactive immune system will be calmed by consuming anti-inflammatory foods. You can not only reduce the symptoms of inflammation by altering your diet, but you can also reverse the progression of existing diseases. There are many different types of autoimmune diseases, including inflammatory bowel disease and Crohn's disease, as well as cardiovascular disease, metabolic disorders such as diabetes and high cholesterol, asthma, and even skin conditions such as eczema. There are also many different types of autoimmune diseases.

Even though more large-scale research is needed, chronic inflammation has been linked to a wide range of serious diseases that affect a large proportion of the general population. Inflammation is linked to a variety of diseases including heart disease, arthritis, diabetes, Alzheimer's disease, depression, and cancer. A number of foods with anti-inflammatory properties have been discovered through experimental studies. A large number of foods and beverages that may cause inflammation have also been found via these investigations.

The correct meals may help you decrease inflammation in your body, delay the progression of existing illnesses, and even reverse them.

Most of the foods associated with inflammation are those which have been labeled as "unhealthy" by the medical community for decades. Consuming excessive amounts of unhealthy foods may lead to weight gain, and being overweight increases the risk of inflammation. But even after taking obesity into consideration, there is an obvious connection between diet and inflammation. A new way of life, and a new you are introduced in Chapter 3.

To regain command of your health, use the tools provided by this website. poisons and chemicals from the body that are produced by the typical diet are eliminated by following an anti-inflammatory diet plan It does not function in an hour or two, as do painkillers, but it does decrease chronic inflammation, increases energy, and does not have the negative effects of painkillers, among other things.

With Chronic Inflammation as a part of your life, are you really living? Many life-altering symptoms accompany chronic inflammation, which makes it difficult to manage. Pain or exhaustion may be making it difficult for you to go out and about. You sit back and watch the world go by, maybe wishing you had spent more time with friends or your grandkids instead of sitting at your computer. It is possible that you may move less even in your own house if your muscles and joints become tight as a result of the inflammation. This often results in weight gain, which only serves to aggravate the discomfort and irritation. You can minimize your pain and swelling in a few of days if you consume anti-inflammatory foods. As soon as the inflammation has decreased, you'll be back on your feet and ready to play with your children or for a stroll with the grandchildren. Simply by eating well and understanding which items to stay away from in your diet, you will notice a boost in your energy and the knowledge that you have been able to make these positive changes in your life.

If you have to give up so many of your favorite foods or follow a very restrictive diet, it may seem challenging, but the advantages outweigh the drawbacks. You can take back control of your life and health by eliminating the foods that trigger inflammation. As a result of following this regimen and exclusively consuming anti-inflammatory meals, you will notice a shift in your taste buds and a decrease in your desire for anti-inflammatory foods. The sweet pastries will soon become a distant memory, and you'll find new favorites. As the inflammation passes, you will notice and feel the difference, and you will never go back.

Many different aspects of your health might be affected by inflammation. It's possible that you were unaware that you weren't feeling well. Possibly, this is quite natural and you were completely unaware of the fact that you might feel stronger and quicker. It's possible that you believed that age or a lack of sleep were to blame for your condition. The anti-inflammatory diet will help to alleviate your exhaustion, and you will be able to sleep better at night once you begin eating it regularly.

However, in order to maintain your health, you should not consider this a diet; rather, you should consider it a new way of eating and living. While eating the appropriate foods might help to decrease inflammation, reverting to your previous eating habits can cause it to return just as rapidly. You must be prepared for this shift in your life circumstances.. It is only you who can make a difference if you are fed up with feeling ill and painful every day.

At this time, there are no long-term drugs available to treat chronic inflammation of the joints. Some of the symptoms of inflammation may be treated with drugs, but many of these medications have adverse effects and may place a burden on your liver and kidneys. You should see your doctor before taking any medication. These side effects might be so distressing that you may be given additional prescriptions to alleviate the discomfort caused by the adverse effects of the first medication. Maintaining control of the illness is a never-ending battle. The high expense of medicine and medical appointments just adds to the frustration and stress of living with this condition.

Change your life for the better by adopting an anti-inflammatory diet, and more crucially by refraining from consuming pro-inflammatory foods, and you'll witness a reduction in medical visits and prescription use over time.

Allowed/avoided meals are discussed in detail in Chapter 4.

A person's immune system may be significantly impacted by their food. Microbiome (bacteria and microorganisms) in the digestive tract plays a role in the regulation of the body's natural defense mechanism. Everything you consume has the potential to either enhance or decrease inflammation....

An adequate intake of fatty acids helps to decrease moderate chronic inflammation while still allowing you to function at your peak performance level. In its most basic form, an anti-inflammatory diet consists of avoiding sugary, processed foods while eating significant quantities of fresh fruits and vegetables, healthy fats from nuts and seeds, unprocessed grains, spices, and herbs. Carbohydrates should also be limited, since they are known to induce a significant amount of swelling.

It is well known that colorful veggies are an excellent source of antioxidants. Eat plenty of colorful veggies and avoid the starchy ones, and you can help your immune system function more effectively and efficiently.

Legumes are a wonderful source of antioxidants and protein, as are many other vegetables. Choose dry beans and soak them overnight before washing and boiling them to save money on chemicals.

Because they include fiber and antioxidants, grains may be beneficial in lowering inflammation if they are consumed in the proper quantities and types. Many individuals, even those who do not have celiac disease, are sensitive to gluten in one way or another. Make sure to pick whole grains that are free of gluten and processed, such as oats, quinoa, barley, and brown rice.

If you are cooking or dressing salads with extra virgin olive oil, you are consuming a healthy fat that is quite beneficial. Extra virgin olive oil includes monounsaturated fat, which is beneficial to the heart, as well as antioxidants and a molecule known as oleocanthal, which has been shown to decrease inflammation in the body.

Many foods should be included in your diet to help decrease chronic inflammation; however, there are other foods that should be avoided in order to assist reduce inflammation as well.

When it comes to inflammation in the western diet, processed foods and sugar are two of the most significant contributors. A lot of the natural fiber and minerals are stripped away from processed meals due to the high degree of refining. The omega-6 fatty acids, trans fats, and saturated fat found in them are all known to increase inflammation in the body.

If you're looking to increase inflammation, sugar is one of the greatest offenders. According to research, it is not only difficult to detect in many meals, but it is also very addictive once consumed. It is for this reason that removing it from your diet will result in a period of withdrawal. Headaches, cravings, and sluggishness are often experienced as a result. Allow yourself some time to allow your body to adjust to this new stage of development. Natural sugars such as honey and agave nectar, as well as refined sweets, cause the body to generate cytokines, which stimulate the immune system and promote inflammation. No natural sugar should be eliminated from your diet completely, but you should aim to consume it just a few times a week and at most once a day at the very most.

The majority of fried meals, particularly deep-fried items, should be avoided as much as possible as well. Their traditional preparation involves the cooking of processed oils or lard, followed by the coating of refined flour, which increases inflammation.

Avoid foods that belong to the nightshade family at all costs. Some individuals are sensitive to night shades, which may have anti-inflammatory properties. If you notice that you have increased inflammation after ingesting one nightshade vegetable, you may want to experiment with substituting other nightshade vegetables in your meals..

Items to include in your diet should be increased, as well as foods to restrict or avoid, as detailed in the following section.. Because this isn't an exhaustive list, keep to the things mentioned before.

Chapter Two

3 week diet plan

Following your improved understanding of what causes chronic inflammation in the body, it is time to begin your new life. Recipes are provided for the following 21 days, which is more than enough to get you through. Cooking Ideas for the Morning Pancakes Made With Coconut Flour

0.25 cup of coconut flour 2 full teaspoons coconut oil (extra virgin coconut oil) 0.25 cup coconut milk Honey (two teaspoons) and organic eggs (three).

A sprinkle of baking powder and pure vanilla extract (0.5 tsp.) Grass-Fed Butter - 0.0625 tablespoons salt to taste maple syrup to taste

To make the honey coconut oil mixture, combine the eggs and coconut oil in a mixing bowl. Stir everything together until it is well combined. Then, while stirring constantly, add the coconut milk and vanilla essence to the egg mixture until well combined.

Gradually incorporate the salt, flour, and baking powder into the batter until well combined. Turn the pancakes out flat if you mix them too much. Stir until everything is properly blended. There should be a few lumps in the mixture, since this is considered desirable.

Now, heat some butter in the pan and pour in the batter using a ladle or measuring cup to make pouring easier.

There will be few bubbles in this batter while it cooks, so be sure to carefully inspect the bottom of your pancake to ensure that it is well cooked before turning it over.

The opposite side of the pancake should be cooked until golden brown, and maple syrup should be drizzled over the top.

Just add another egg if you aren't satisfied with the consistency of your pancakes.

2 persons may eat up to 8 pancakes (depending on size).

Pie made of sweet potatoes, spinach, and kale.

1 large sweet potato, 2 medium-sized sweet potatoes 0.5 cup of finely diced spinach

Chop and stem the kale to make a cup. 1. Finely sliced white onion (0.2 cup) 0.5 teaspoon table salt

1 teaspoon of cumin 3 tablespoons of avocado oil

Full Fat Coconut Milk - 2 tablespoons Garlic powder (optional) 1 teaspoon

Before you begin, peel and chop the potatoes into 12 inch cubes (about).

Using a steamer basket, steam the potatoes until they are cooked in a saucepan with about an inch of water in it.

Using a slotted spoon, transfer the sweet potatoes to a bowl. Using a blender, mix in the milk until there are no lumps left.

In a large mixing bowl, combine the kale with the onion and spinach along with cumin, sea salt, and garlic. Everything should be well blended. Using the ingredients, shape 6-8 separate patties.

Fry all patties until they are browned on all sides in avocado oil.

It serves 6 people.

Chia Pudding With Turmeric and Chocolate

Ingredients: Coconut Milk (one can), Chia Seeds (three-quarter cup), and Vanilla Extract

Cocoa Powder (without sugar):.25 cup cinnamon (approximately 5 teaspoons)

Raw Honey (0.5 tablespoons) - 1 teaspoon ground turmeric .5 teaspoons of vanilla extract

Choose your own toppings from nuts to fruits to shredded coconut to serve with your dish!

Place the vanilla, honey, turmeric, cinnamon, cocoa powder, chia seeds, and milk in a blender and mix until smooth, about 30 seconds. Serve immediately.

Stir often and refrigerate for at least 4 hours, or until the mixture has thickened. Garnish with chosen items after putting everything in a dish.

Allow to cool before serving.

This recipe serves two people.

During the night, I make Mango Turmeric Oatmeal.

Breakfast cereal made from oats

milk 5 quarts 2 tablespoons kefir or Greek yogurt,.5 cup almond milk, 1 cup maple syrup, and 2 teaspoons vanilla extract 25 tablespoons of ground turmeric Spices: Ground Cinnamon-.25 teaspoons Ground Cardamom-1 teaspoon Chia seeds-1 teaspoon Ground Ginger-1 tablespoon Ground Cardamom-.25 teaspoons

a half-cup of finely diced mango (fresh or frozen)

Add 14 cup rolled oats, 14 cup milk kefir or Greek yogurt, and 14 cup almond milk to two mason jars and shake vigorously until well combined and smooth.

In each glass, divide the chia seeds and spices evenly. Stir until the ingredients are well combined. The mango chunks should be placed in the glasses.

Refrigerate the jars for at least one night.

You may drink it cold directly from the glass, or pour it into a bowl and heat it in the microwave.

This recipe serves two people.

Casserole with Maple Rice and Pumpkin

Granulated rice is a kind of grain that has a nutty taste to it.

1.5 tablespoons vanilla extract per 5 cup of vanilla extract 2 tablespoons of pure maple syrup cinnamon (a pinch or two)

a pinch of salt (but not too much) (optional)

Fruits such as pears, plums, berries, and cherries that have been cut into slices

Start by preheating the oven to 400 degrees Fahrenheit and leaving it on for a few minutes.

Using a medium-high heat, bring the rice and one cup of water to a boil in a small pot. Meanwhile, while the food is cooking, mix in the cinnamon and vanilla essence until everything is well incorporated.

Turn lower the heat to medium/low and cover the saucepan with a lid. Allow for 10-15 minutes of simmering time till the rice is cooked.

Rice should be stirred well before being divided into two oven-safe serving dishes. Sprinkle salt to taste over the tops of each bowl, then drizzle with maple syrup and add sliced fruit as desired.

Cook the rice bowls for 10-15 minutes, or until the syrup begins to boil and the fruit topping begins to caramelize.

Serve as soon as possible after preparing it.

This recipe serves two people.

For dinner, I made pecan banana oatmeal.

Classic oatmeal: 1 cup ripe bananas, 2 cups almond milk, and 1.5 cups plain Greek yogurt (old-fashioned).

Tablespoons of 25 cup Chia seeds 2 teaspoons of honey

- 2 tablespoons unsweetened coconut flakes - 2 teaspoons roasted vanilla extract

.25 tablespoons sea salt (in flakes).

The ingredients for the dessert are banana slices, fig halves, roasted nuts, pomegranate seeds, and honey. Using a mixer, combine all of the ingredients (except fruit and nuts for serving).

Combine all of the ingredients well to ensure that they are well-mixed and uniform. Make two bowls or glasses out of the mixture and divide it equally.

Refrigerate overnight or for at least 6 hours after covering the bowls with a lid. Reheat the mixture if necessary once it has been well mixed.

The banana slices, figs, toasted nuts, and pomegranate seeds are placed on top of the chia pudding mixture. Enjoy with a drizzle of honey.

This recipe serves two people.

Portion of cereal for breakfast

2 cups soaked grains (such as amaranth or buckwheat) - 1 cup nut milk or coconut water - 2.5 cups

(1) Cinnamon sprig 2 star anise (whole cloves) (optional) the absence of one pod

A variety of fresh fruits, including but not limited to cranberries and blackberries, apples and pears, or any other fruit of your choosing sweetener made from maple trees (optional)

In a small saucepan, combine the grains, coconut water or nut milk, and spices and cook over medium-high heat until the grains are a brittle consistency.

As soon as the grains begin to boil, cover the saucepan with a lid and reduce the heat to medium. Pour in enough water to cover the grains and bring them to a boil.

Remove the pan from the heat and toss out all the spices. Prepare the fruit of your choosing, drizzle it with maple syrup, and garnish with it.

This recipe serves two people.

Hash browns with turkey and apple

For the meat, use the following ingredients.

Grounded Turkey - 1 lb Cinnamon-5 teaspoons Dried Thyme-5 teaspoons Coconut Oil-1 tablespoon sea salt to taste Grounded Turkey - 1 lb Cinnamon-5 teaspoons Dried Thyme-5 teaspoons Coconut Oil-1 tablespoon sea salt to taste

Here's all you need to know about it:

carrots, 5 cups shredded coconut oil, 5 tablespoons zucchini, 1 big onion, peeled, cored, and cut into small cubes 1 large apple, peeled, cored, and cut into cubes 2-cups frozen butternut squash cubes (chopped)

2 cups of spinach

.75 tablespoons of ginger powder 1-tablespoon cinnamon-.5-tablespoon garlic powder 5-tablespoons dried thyme in place of the turmeric When using sea salt, use 5 teaspoons.

On a medium-high stove, heat the coconut oil until it is hot. Prepare the turkey and roast it until it is golden brown, around 30 minutes.

Season the ground turkey with a 12 teaspoon mixture of cinnamon, thyme, and salt. Transfer to a platter once you've combined the ingredients.

Continue to cook the onion until it is tender in the same pan with the remaining coconut oil.

Then, heat for another 4.5 minutes while the apple, carrot, zucchini, and frozen squash cook in the pan. Mix in the spinach when the veggies have softened.

the plant will eventually die

In a large mixing bowl, thoroughly combine the cooked turkey and additional seasonings. If necessary, season with salt before turning off the burner.

Take advantage of the hash while it's still hot and fresh, or store it in the refrigerator for later use.

Hash will keep in the fridge for about 5-6 days if it is stored in a firmly sealed container.

It serves 5 people.

Chapter Three

Nutritional Bar with Chia Seeds.

Pitted dates, 1.5 cup packed raw walnut pieces, 1.25 cups raw cocoa powder, and .33 cup whole chia seeds are all you need to make this delicious dessert.

Unsweetened coconut (about 5 cups)

Oatmeal (whole) in a quantity of 5 cups (crushed).

5.25 cups Pure Vanilla Extract - 1 teaspoon Dark chocolate -.5 cup coarsely chopped Sea Salt-.25 teaspoons

Puree the dates until they are thick and smooth in a food processor. Using your blender, mix the raw walnut bits until smooth.

Toss in the rest of the ingredients until everything is well distributed.

To make the dough-like consistency, place a piece of parchment paper on top of the baking pan, leaving a few inches above the pan to allow for easy removal, and press the dough firmly into the pan, making sure to get into all of the corners and edges.

Place the baking pan in the freezer for at least 4 hours or overnight. Exit the freezer and carefully pull out the lump of dough that has been frozen in place. Using a knife, cut the dough into 14 bars.

Refrigeration is recommended for storing in an airtight container.

This recipe serves 14 people.

Custard Pudding with Bananas and Chia

1-2 large Chia Seeds (banana)

5 cup unsweetened almond milk - 2 teaspoons raw honey - 5 cup unsweetened coconut milk 1 tablespoon cocoa powder Vanilla extract (0.5 teaspoon)

Interfere:\sBanana

- 1 cup large dark chocolate chips - 2 tablespoons cocoa nibs - 2 teaspoons vanilla bean powder

Mix one banana and the chia seeds together in a medium-sized mixing bowl until well blended. whisking constantly, until there are no lumps, add the almond milk and vanilla extract.

Half of your mixture should be placed in an airtight container with a tight-fitting lid.

Whisk in the honey (or maple syrup) and cocoa powder to the remaining half of the batter until everything is thoroughly blended. (Optional)

Immediately transfer the cocoa mixture to a second container and seal it tightly. In a refrigerator overnight or for at least 4 hours, place the two containers of ingredients.

Prepare three separate containers by layering the two puddings and all of the ingredients equally on top of them. This dish may be kept in the refrigerator for up to 5 days in an airtight bowl.

3 servings are provided by this recipe!

Porridge

1. Walnut or Pecan halves - 0.25 cup, finely chopped 0.25 cup toasted unsweetened coconut (unsweetened is preferred).

2 teaspoons of hemp seeds 1 cup unsweetened almond milk - 0.75 cup 2 teaspoons of whole chia seeds 1 cup coconut milk - 0.25 cup coconut oil - 3 teaspoones 0.25 cup Almond butter 0.25 cup Cinnamon 0.5 teaspoon Turmeric powder 0.5 teaspoon

0.0625 teaspoons of black pepper

Using a hot pan, toast the chopped walnuts (or pecans), coconut, and hemp seeds until fragrant, approximately 1-2 minutes total. In order to prevent the coconut and nuts from burning, turn them over many times.

Using a slotted spoon, transfer the nuts to a dish and put away until no longer warm.

Melt the almond and coconut milks together in a small saucepan over medium heat until warm. Remove the milk from the fire as soon as it is warm but not boiling.

Toss the cinnamon and turmeric powder together in a small bowl and stir into the milk, along with the coconut oil, almond butter, chia seeds, and black pepper to taste. Remove from heat and put aside to cool for 5-8 minutes, or until the mixture is thoroughly mixed.

Add about half of the seed and nut mixture and stir well..

Separate the porridge into two serving dishes and top with the leftover toasted mixture.

In a firmly covered dish, preserve in the refrigerator for up to 3 days, or serve immediately. When keeping the leftover toasted mixture, keep it separate and at room temperature until needed. To keep it crispy, add it immediately before serving.

This recipe serves two people.

Cake Muffins made with Sweet Potatoes

1 boiled sweet potato-1 small organic egg-1 brown rice flour - 1 cup Coconut milk - 0.75 cup coconut flour -0.25 cup Pure Maple Syrup - 0.5 cup baking soda-3 teaspoons olive oil-6 teaspoons salt-1/2 teaspoon cinnamon powder-3 teaspoons ginger powder -1 teaspoon Turmeric powder - 1 teaspoon toasted walnuts 0.125 tablespoons of ground cloves 0.125 teaspoon freshly ground nutmeg

Set the oven to 400 degrees Fahrenheit and bake for 30 minutes.

Cut in half the cooked sweet potato once it has been allowed to cool. Using a spoon, scoop out the sweet potato's inside and place it in a mixing dish.

Combine the sweet potato with the egg, olive oil, maple syrup, and coconut milk until it is smooth.

In a separate dish, combine all of the additional ingredients and stir them into the sweet potatoes until they are well combined. Everything should be well blended.

Preparation: Grease a muffin tray and fill each one approximately two-thirds of the way with batter. inferior

It serves 12 people.

In a baking dish, bake eggs with turmeric.

8-10 big organic eggs (organic if possible). 0.5 cup unsweetened almond milk 0.25 teaspoon black pepper

0.75 teaspoon ground turmeric 1 tsp. cumin powder

0.25 teaspoon sea salt

@ least 2 baking pans "a long way (about 18" x 26" or a 9" x 13" baking pan) Avocado, salsa, cilantro, and other optional garnishes

Pre-heat the oven to 350 degrees Fahrenheit by turning on the oven.

Using a medium-sized mixing bowl, whisk together the eggs, milk, and spices until well combined. The tray should be lightly oiled (or the baking pan).

Pour the eggs onto the baking sheet with care and watch them cook.

Using a timer, bake the eggs for 10-12 minutes at 350 degrees. Once the eggs have begun to set, take the pan from the oven and gently mix the eggs without spilling them, then place the pan back in the oven to finish setting..

For a firmer set, bake the eggs for another 8 to 10 minutes, or until they are set. The eggs should be taken out of the oven and whisked a second time.

As a garnish, you may use paprika, cilantro, avocado, or whatever else you choose.

A chilled, airtight container may be used to preserve baked eggs for up to 4 days after they are baked.

If you want to utilize the eggs to make a quick sandwich, you may bake them for 15 to 17 minutes without stirring them, then cut them into squares.

This recipe serves 5 to 6 people.

Mallow Muffins with Berries and Turmeric

Whole Wheat Flour (1.333 cup):

In addition to greasing the cans, use 0.5 cup of coconut oil. Flour for All Purposes- 8 oz.

Unsweetened Almond Milk - 8 oz (0.5 cup) Raw sugar (0.5 cup)

0.33 cup + 1 tablespoon pure maple syrup 1 teaspoon of baking soda

a teaspoon of baking powder .5 tablespoons of ground turmeric. 0.5 teaspoon salt

0.5 teaspoon cardamom

0.5 teaspoon of pure vanilla bean extract

Whisked apple cider vinegar - 2 teaspoons Organic eggs - 2 at room temperature

1 cup toasted chopped walnuts

Raspberry puree (fresh or frozen) 1 cup 1 tablespoon of chia seeds

One-cup of blueberries, either fresh or frozen. 3-tablespoons of oatmeal

Preheat the oven to 400 degrees Fahrenheit (200 degrees Celsius). Prepare 2 muffin tins by brushing them with coconut oil..

Using a whisk, combine the flours (all-purpose, whole wheat, salt), baking powder, baking soda, turmeric, and cardamom in a large mixing bowl.

Meanwhile, in a separate dish, whisk together the sugar and coconut oil for 1 to 2 minutes, or until the sugar has partially dissolved. Then, combine the maple syrup, almond milk, eggs, vanilla extract, and apple cider vinegar in a large mixing bowl until everything is thoroughly blended.

In a separate bowl, whisk together the dry ingredients and the egg mixture until fully incorporated but with some tiny lumps still visible. In a large mixing bowl, gently fold in the berries, walnuts, and chia seeds until evenly distributed.

Fill the muffin liners approximately two-thirds of the way filled with the batter, then pour some oats and the leftover raw sugar onto the muffin liners to finish them up.

Allow for about 5 minutes of resting time for the muffin batter.

Bake the muffins for 13 to 15 minutes, depending on their size. Insert a wooden toothpick right into the middle of one of the muffins to see whether they are finished baking. When you take it out, it should be clean, which means the muffins are finished. After 10 minutes in the pan, remove the muffins from the tin and set them on a wire rack to cool completely.

There are 18 servings in this recipe!

Chapter Four

Carrot Pancakes with Cream Cheese Frosting

Coconut flour (0.5 cup) Very ripe banana (0.25) Pumpkin puree (0.25) Coconut oil (3.5 teaspoons) melted coconut oil 4 organic eggs (0.5 teaspoon ground cinnamon, 0.125 teaspoon black pepper) 1.75 tablespoons frying oil of your choice 2.75 teaspoons pure vanilla extract 3.25 teaspoons ground turmeric

In a blender, combine all of the ingredients except the cooking oil and process until smooth, scraping the sides of the blender occasionally to ensure that everything is well blended.

Enable for a few minutes of resting time to allow the coconut flour to absorb the liquid. Cooking oil should be heated in a pan on a medium-high burner before you start.

The batter should be carefully poured into the pan after it has reached a temperature of around 325 degrees F "with respect to circumference Remove from the oven and bake for another minute or two, or until gently browned on the opposite side.

Served with maple syrup, honey, or fresh fruit on the side for a festive touch,

10-12 tiny pancakes may be made using this recipe!

Soups and stews are some of the most popular dishes in the United States today.

Soup made with vegetables

3 or 4 cups of filtered water is recommended.

3 cups of chopped cauliflower florets

Canned Great Northern Beans (about 15 ounces), drained, and rinsed 7 ounces of Shirataki Noodles (drained from package)

Chop up one bunch of kale.

vegetable stock - 1 packet of 32 oz vegetable stock 1 medium carrot, finely chopped 1 onion, diced 1 tablespoon celery, finely chopped - 1 tablespoon of olive oil 1 tablespoon of ground turmeric 0.5 teaspoon of ground ginger

2 teaspoons minced garlic 0.25 teaspoon freshly ground cayenne pepper 1-tablespoon of salt

Add a dash of cracked black pepper to taste.

Using a medium-low burner, warm the oil up.

Continue to cook while stirring the onion until it is lightly browned.

Afterwards, the celery and carrots are added to the pot and allowed to soften while constantly stirring.

Using a large mixing bowl, evenly distribute the turmeric, ginger, garlic, and cayenne pepper over the vegetables. Prepare the dish for about 1 minute, or until the flavors have melded completely.

Toss in the water and broth along with the salt and pepper until everything is well-combined.

Cook over medium heat until the pot is just simmering, then reduce the heat to low.

Cover the pot with a lid and cook for another 15 minutes. Reduce heat to low and simmer for 10 to 15 minutes or until the cauliflower is tender.

Following a few minutes of cooking, remove the cauliflower and set it aside to cool slightly before adding the beans, kale, and pasta to the pot. Cook until the kale has wilted slightly, then remove from the heat and serve immediately.

This recipe serves four people.

a soup made with broccoli and cream

3 tablespoons of ghee or grass-fed butter 0.5 cup diced white onion

Two minced or sliced garlic cloves 3-cups of homemade chicken or bone broth 8 oz. of coconut cream

1 pound broccoli florets Leek-1 is a fictional character created by the fictional character Leek in the year 2000. (white only) as needed, season with pepper and salt

On a medium-high burner, melt the ghee until it is hot.

The onion should be soft and translucent after 1 to 2 minutes of sautéing in ghee. Stirring frequently, cook for 1 minute until the garlic and onion are fragrant.

Sprinkle salt and pepper over the leeks and broccoli after they have been carefully added to the saucepan.

Turn down the heat to low and allow the broccoli to simmer for about 20 minutes, or until the broccoli is tender.

When the rice is done, add the coconut milk to the pot and mix well. Allow the milk to come to room temperature before transferring it to a food processor with the remaining ingredients from the pan. The soup should be free of lumps and thoroughly combined at this point.

Prepare and serve immediately in individual serving bowls, if desired. Hot food should be served.

4-6 people can be fed from this recipe.

Bisque de crevettes de crevettes de crevettes de crevettes

1-large jar of roasted red peppers

Light 15 oz. of coconut cream 2 quarts of chicken broth 1 teaspoon of finely chopped garlic 0.25 cup barbecue sauce 0.75 cup finely chopped olive oil-3 tablespoons water-3 teaspoons shallots

2 tablespoons of tapioca or potato starch 0.25 teaspoon ground mustard

0.5 teaspoon cayenne pepper

1 teaspoon of red pepper flakes Ginger powder, a pinch of it should be garnished with freshly chopped coriander

Pre-heat the oven to 475 degrees Fahrenheit and bake the cake.

On a baking sheet, roast the red peppers for 10 minutes, until they are soft. Fry for another 5 to 10 minutes after flipping the peppers.

During the final 2 to 3 minutes of cooking, grill the peppers over low heat. Remove the baking sheet from the oven and set it aside to cool completely.

As soon as the peppers have cooled, they can be peeled, and then the stalks may be cut away and the seeds can be removed.

The garlic and shallots should be sautéed in olive oil in a medium-sized pot over medium heat until soft. Once the flavors have established, add the water and peeled shrimp to the saucepan and bring it to a boil again.

Allow the shrimp to cook until pink, approximately 6 to 8 minutes for medium-sized shrimp, over medium-high heat.

Stir in the black pepper and salt until everything is well-coordinated.

As soon as the shrimp are finished, remove them from the saucepan and put them aside.

Stir well after adding the coconut milk, broth, starch, and spices to the pot. Cook for about 5 minutes after combining the ingredients in a saucepan.

In a blender, mix the roasted peppers, liquid, and BBQ sauce until smooth.

Cook until the bisque comes to a mild boil in the same pot as before. Reduce the heat to "on" (simmer) and let it cook for 10 to 20 minutes before re-incorporating the shrimp into the pot of broth. Re-add the shrimp to the soup and stir well.

Fresh coriander should be garnished on the plate soon after serving.

This recipe serves four people.

Soup de poulet à la Mexicana

One 14-ounce can of Fire Roasted Plum Tomatoes 1 pound boneless, skinless chicken breast

peppers - 1 sliced red pepper 1.5 cups of chicken broth - 1 cup of half and half.

Cream 1/2 cup shredded cheese, room temp. Cheddar 1 cup shredded cheese 2 tablespoons extra-virgin olive oil

2 cloves of minced garlic 1 big diced onion 1 teaspoon paprika 1 teaspoon paprika

1. 5 tablespoons of cumin powder 0.5 tablespoon Chipotle Chili Powder 1 teaspoon salt, to taste, dried oregano

should be garnished with freshly chopped coriander

On a medium-high burner, heat the oil until it is hot.

The onion and garlic should be sautéed after the oil is hot, turning regularly to prevent them from burning. As soon as they are soft, remove them from the heat.

Chicken breasts, fire roasted tomatoes, onions, garlic, all of the spices, and chicken stock are placed in a prepared pot and brought to a simmer. Squeeze some lemon juice over the top.

Cook on high for 3 hours in a slow cooker to ensure even heating.

Chop peppers and combine them with the cream cheese and half and half. Add the shredded cheese on top if desired. Cook for a further 20 minutes to half an hour, or until the cheese has melted, before covering with foil.

With two forks, shred the chicken and mix it back in until everything is thoroughly blended. Fresh cilantro or avocado and sour cream may be added to the soup after it is served.

It serves 5 people.

Soup with miso

4-cups of ice

Cooking Instructions: 1 cup Shiitake Mushrooms-6 Dried Potatoes-2 big diced Kombu-1 piece Yellow Onion-1 finely chopped Firm Tofu - 1 block diced Carrot-1 thinly sliced Brown miso paste (about 2 tablespoons) 2 teaspoons of dried Wakame 1 tablespoon of white miso paste As a garnish, finely chopped green onion.

For about 10 minutes, soak the dried shiitake mushrooms in warm water. Drain the mushrooms and keep the liquid aside for later use in a separate bowl. Mushrooms should be sliced thinly.

A big saucepan should hold the water and potatoes. Over medium-high heat, bring the water to a boil.

Reduce the heat on the stove to a low setting and carry on cooking. As soon as the potatoes are readily pierced with a fork, add the yellow onion, fish stock, kombu, tofu, slices of shiitake mushrooms, carrots, and wakame to the saucepan and continue to boil until all of the veggies are tender.

Using a blender, puree the soup until all of the miso paste is thoroughly incorporated. Using the spring onions as a garnish for the soup, serve it.

This recipe serves two people.

a stew made with red lentils and pumpkin

4 cups of broth 3 cooked cups of butternut squash, 1 cup red lentils, and any greens of your choosing 3 garlic cloves, finely chopped Curry powder 1 teaspoon extra virgin olive oil 2 tblsp. Sweet Onion - 1 chopped Onion - 1 chopped Onion to taste with freshly grated ginger As required, season with black pepper and salt.

Preparation time: 5 minutes in a big saucepan over low-medium heat with the olive oil, diced onion, and garlic.

Sauté for 2 to 3 minutes, until the curry powder is well incorporated. Pour in the broth slowly, stirring constantly, and bring the red lentil stew to a boil, stirring often.

Once the stew starts to boil, reduce the heat on the stove to low and continue to simmer for around 10 minutes more.

Cook for 5 to 8 minutes over medium-high heat, stirring occasionally, until the pumpkin and veggies are soft. Season with ginger, pepper, and salt to taste after cooking for 5 to 8 minutes.

This recipe serves four people.

Chili made with turkey

Black Beans - 30 ounces canned black beans, drained and rinsed Lean ground turkey - 1 pound red peppers - 1 chopped Tomato Sauce - 30 ounces canned tomato sauce 15 ounces canned diced tomatoes (small diced) 1 yellow pepper (chopped) 15 ounces canned diced tomatoes 1 cup frozen corn Red Kidney Beans (30 ounces, canned, washed and rinsed) 1 cup frozen corn sliced Jalapeno peppers - 1 jar (16 oz) onion - 1 medium diced olive oil - 3 teaspoons cumin - 3 teaspoons chili powder - 2 tablespoons pepper and salt - 1 jar (16 oz) tomato sauce

Avocado, shredded cheese, sour cream, and green onions are optional toppings. Medium-high heat is used to heat the olive oil.

Preheat a skillet over medium heat until the turkey is browned, then transfer to a slow cooker pot.

Add the tomato sauce, beans, onions, jalapenos, peppers, diced tomatoes, cumin, chili powder, and corn to a slow cooker and season with salt and pepper to taste.

Stir the ingredients together in a saucepan and cover with a lid while cooking. Bake at 350°F for 6 hours or at 400°F for 4 hours on low setting.

Makes plenty for eight people to share it.

Chapter Five

Beef stew with sweet potatoes and carrots

Beef broth (1.5 cup) - 3 pounds ground beef

Tomatoes (diced) - 1 can (14 oz) diced tomatoes 1. Tomato paste - 0.25 cup 2. Almond flour - 0.33 cup 3. Onion - 1 big minced garlic clove 4. Almond flour - 0.33 cup 5.

3 cups sweet potato, peeled and cut into cubes about 2 inches in size Half a pound of baby potatoes (0.666 pounds)

Red bell peppers - 2 large, thinly sliced Carrots 1.25 cup beef stock cubes, seeded and diced 2.25 cup crushed olive oil 1-tablespoon of salt Garnish: 4 tablespoons fresh chopped parsley, freshly ground black pepper, 0.5 teaspoon bay leaves, and 2 teaspoons paprika. Pepper and salt should be sprinkled on both sides of the steak.

1 tablespoon oil is heated over medium-high heat in a skillet.

The meat should be seared for 2 to 3 minutes each side, or until it has browned. Make sure to fry in batches so that the pan does not get overcrowded, and add more oil if necessary.

The meat should be browned before being placed in the slow cooker saucepan.

The onion should only be softened after it has been sautéed in the remaining oil. Continue to cook for approximately 60 seconds after adding the garlic to the onions.

Along with the steak, put in the garlic and onions in a saucepan.

Stir in the flour until the meat, garlic, and onion are well coated with the flour. (Optional) Except for the bay leaves and parsley, combine all of the other ingredients. In a large mixing bowl, whisk together the ingredients until thoroughly combined, then add the bay leaves.

Cover with a cover and cook on high for 4 to 6 hours or on low for 8 to 10 hours, until the vegetables are tender. Season with salt and pepper to taste, then garnish with parsley if desired. -

Makes plenty for eight people to share it.

A tomato-kale-quinoa soup topped with feta cheese.

4 quarts of vegetable stock

Prepare quinoa according to package directions: 1 cup uncooked and drained water-2 cups

great northern beans (from a 15-ounce can, washed and drained): 14.5 ounces each of small diced tomatoes from 2 cans

3 cloves of garlic, minced onion, diced, 0.5 tbsp. dried basil

0.25 tsp of dried rosemary 0.5 teaspoon dried oregano 1 bunch of chopped kale (with the stems removed) 2 bay leaves 0.25 teaspoon dried thyme

peppercorns and sea salt, freshly ground

In a slow cooker, combine the quinoa, tomatoes, beans, garlic, onion, rosemary, basil, oregano, bay leaves, and thyme. Cook on low for 8 hours or on high for 4 hours. Serve immediately.

Stir in the broth and water until everything is well-combined, then serve. If necessary, season with salt and pepper.

Place the cover on the pot of your slow cooker and set it to low heat for 7 to 8 hours or high heat for 3 to 4 hours to cook.

In a separate bowl, combine the kale and toss until it is wilted before serving.

Kale Turkey Meatball Soup yields 8 servings.

One 15-ounce can of great northern beans that has been drained and rinsed 8 cups of vegetable broth

0.25 cup of almond milk 0.5 cup grated Parmesan cheese 2 pieces of bread

Peeled and cut carrots (two pounds) 0.5 cup chopped yellow onion turkey breast, 1 lb. lean ground turkey 4 cups chopped kale

Beaten Organic Egg No. 1 Organic Egg No. 1 2 cloves of garlic, peeled and chopped finely sliced shallot (one medium-sized) 0.5 teaspoon ground nutmeg

0.25 tsp. crushed red pepper flakes 1-tablespoon dried oregano

1 tablespoon extra-virgin olive oil.

2 tablespoons finely chopped Italian parsley.

Prepare a medium-sized basin of milk and set the bread slices in it to soak.

Afterwards, combine all of the ingredients by gently mixing with your hands until everything is well-combined (garlic, turkey, nutmeg, shallot, pepper, red pepper flakes, oregano, cheese, parsley, egg, and salt).

Using your hands, form 12" balls with the meat mixture.

Preheat a large pan over medium-high heat and sear the meatballs for approximately 1 to 2 minutes each side, depending on how big they are.

Remove the meatballs from the pan and place them on a plate to cool completely.

Then add the carrots and beans to the pot with the greens and the onions.

Cover and simmer on low for 4 hours, until the meatballs float to the top of the kale in the slow cooker, then remove the lid and cook for another 4 hours.

Sprinkle grated parmesan and fresh parsley on top of each bowl of soup before serving it.

Makes plenty for eight people to share it.

a soup made with broccoli

 Broccolli with florets (about 8 cup total). 6 cups of broth

 Chopped leek (four cups) 2 tbsp. of melted butter 1 cup fresh ginger, minced 1 teaspoon of ground turmeric 1-tablespoon of salt

 1 tablespoon sesame seed oil

 one or two grinds of freshly ground black pepper

 Over medium heat, melt the butter in a large pan.

 Cook the leeks, stirring occasionally, for approximately 8 minutes, or until they are soft and translucent.

 Slow-cook the leeks in the broth until they are soft. Stir in the ginger and broccoli as well as the turmeric, sesame oil, and salt until the leeks are tender.

 Cook on low for 3 to 4 hours, or until the broccoli is soft, covered with a tight fitting pot lid. Smooth and creamy is the result of blending the soup.

 There should be enough for 6-8 people to share this recipe.

 Soup with Zoodles and Chicken

 Boiled and diced chicken meat (four cups), 6 cups of low-sodium chicken stock 2 medium-size onions, diced

 Chopped garlic (six cloves)

Peeled and sliced carrots (three big ones), 2 medium-sized Zucchini or Zoodles (from a package). Chopped celery (three big stalks plus leaves) 2 tablespoons of avocado oil

1 tablespoon of ground turmeric 3 bay leaves, 1 teaspoon dried rosemary, a pinch of salt and pepper 1 teaspoon of dried sage Sea salt - 1 teaspoon (or more to taste) dried thyme - 1 teaspoon (1 teaspoon dried thyme)

The avocado oil should be heated over medium-high heat in a large saucepan.

Stir in the turmeric for approximately 90 seconds in the oil to enable the flavor to emerge. Cook, stirring occasionally, until the onions and garlic are just beginning to become transparent.

Continue to simmer for a few more minutes until the celery and carrots are just starting to soften. Season with sea salt and pepper after adding the broth and chicken. Saute until the chicken is done.

To make the soup, bring it to a boil, then decrease the heat to low and let it simmer, covered, for 25-30 minutes.

Cook for another 15 minutes or until vegetables are soft and the chicken is coming apart. Taste and adjust seasoning if necessary.

Make zucchini noodles using a spiralizer fitted with a pasta attachment. Zucchini noodles should be sliced into 2" to 3" pieces using a knife. In the absence of a spiralizer, pre-packaged Zoodles may be purchased.

Remove the pot of soup from the heat and discard the bay leaves before continuing.

Stir in the zoodles until everything is well-combined and evenly distributed. Because of the remaining heat from the soup, the zoodles are cooked until they are soft. Enjoy!

There should be enough for 6-8 people to share this recipe.

a soup made with cauliflower and turmeric

Cut 1 medium-sized head of cauliflower into bits before serving. 2 and a half cups unsweetened almond/cashew milk blend 2 cups of vegetable stock

1.5 cups red lentils 1 medium shallot, quartered 0.5 cup shallot 3 or 4 cloves of garlic 1 teaspoon extra-virgin olive oil-6 tablespoons ground turmeric 0.5 teaspoon table salt

1 teaspoon of cumin powder

Add garnishes such as peppercorns, lime wedges, fresh herbs, or other seasonal ingredients. Set the oven to 425 degrees Fahrenheit and bake for 30 minutes.

Olive oil should be drizzled over the cauliflower, shallots, and garlic in a large mixing bowl to prevent sticking.

15 minutes of roasting the vegetables on a large baking sheet Roast for another 15 minutes after flipping the vegetables.

In a large saucepan, combine all of the vegetables after they have been roasted.

Add 2 cups of milk, the broth, and the lentils one at a time, whisking constantly. Combine thoroughly until everything is well-combined................. Bring the soup to a boil, then cover it with a tight fitting lid. Reduce the heat to low and simmer for 20 minutes.

Using a blender, blend the soup together. Using a whisk, thoroughly combine the soup and remove any lumps before adding the remaining milk and garnishing with your favorite garnishes.

This recipe serves four people.

Chicken Soup with Lemon and Cream

6 cups of bone broth

4 cups cooked and shredded chicken (optional). onion - 1 cup, diced - olive oil 0.5 cup Kale 1 Bundle Lemon Juice - 2 tablespoons, freshly squeezed Lemon - 3 teaspoons, kosher salt

Rinse and dry the kale, then divide it into two piles and cut it into 12 inch strips. Set the kale aside.

In a blender, combine 2 cups broth, 1 tablespoon olive oil, and 1 tablespoon diced onion. Blend on high for 1-2 minutes, or until the mixture is smooth and homogenous.

In a medium-sized saucepan, combine the contents of your blender with the remaining 4 cups of broth. Then, along with the fresh lemon juice, combine the shredded chicken, chopped kale, and the zest of all three lemons in a large mixing bowl. Squeeze some lemon juice over the top.

6 hours on low heat is sufficient time to cook the soup.

It serves 6 people.

Soup of vegetables with a variety of textures and flavors

4-cups of ice

2 cups of diced butternut squash 1 cup of diced red peppers 1 celery stalk (cut into pieces) 2 cups diced

1 cup of diced carrots 1 cup of diced Zucchini 1 cup finely diced red onions

Cut 1 cup of spring onions finely and reserve the rest for garnishing. Cup celery leaves (approximately 1 cup

3 large cloves of garlic salt to taste - lemon juice - 2 tablespoons

A large saucepan should have enough water to cover all the vegetables. Add the red bell pepper (with seeds), butternut squash (with seeds), zucchini (with seeds), red onion (with spring onion), celery leaves (with stalks), and garlic cloves.

Once you've brought the water to a boil, turn the heat down to a medium level. Simmer the ingredients for about 40 minutes, or until the vegetables are tender, depending on the size of the vegetables.

After that, incorporate the lemon juice thoroughly. Squeeze some lemon juice over the top.

This recipe serves four people. Soups, salads, and side dishes are all available. Salad de beets (beetroot)

salad dressing with sweet kale (with Nut and Seed Packet) 24 ounce bag (optional). cooked, peeled, and diced beetroot (16 ounces),

Fresh blueberries (1.5 cups) –

Dressing made with turmeric: 0.33 cup extra virgin olive oil, 1 tablespoon lemon juice, 2 tablespoons apple cider vinegar 1 teaspoon of turmeric

1 teaspoon freshly grated ginger, 1 clove freshly grated garlic

0.5 teaspoon table salt

0.25 tsp. freshly grated black pepper

The dressing is made by combining all of the ingredients. To make a smoother dressing, shake or puree the ingredients together.

Divide the kale salad between two bowls and top with the blueberries, beetroot, and nut and seed mixture.

The turmeric dressing should be drizzled over the salad.

4-6 people may be fed using this recipe.

Tuna salad is a dish that is popular in the United Kingdom.

To make cannellini beans, rinse and drain one 15-ounce can of cannellini beans.

Tuna 1 can of Packed in Oil (Use 2 cans if you want to make the salad with tuna) 0.5 cup finely diced onions

1 cup finely chopped parsley (about 0.25 cup)

1 or 2 tablespoons of fresh herbs, such as basil. Depending on personal preference, extra virgin olive oil

depending on your personal preference

peppercorns freshly ground to your liking Depending on your preference, red wine vinegar

The canned beans should be rinsed and drained before cooking. Pour the ingredients into a medium-sized mixing bowl and combine well. In a large mixing bowl, combine the tuna and beans. Do not drain the tuna and beans; instead, combine them with the onions. In a separate bowl, combine the chopped parsley and basil.

Drizzle the dish with olive oil and red wine vinegar after seasoning with salt and pepper. Enjoy!

This recipe serves two people.

A quinoa salad is a delicious and nutritious dish.

Chapter Six

To make the salad, cook two cups of quinoa.

Recipe for Roasted Almonds: 0.33 cup raw almonds - 1 teaspoon low sodium Tamari - 1 teaspoon coconut oil - 1 teaspoon sea salt (or to taste) - 0.25 teaspoon roasted almonds

Chickpeas (cooked, rinsed, and drained): 2 cups 1 cucumber, diced (about 2 cups).
  peeled and chopped Eddamame: 1 cup
  1/2 a cup shredded purple cabbage 1 cup of roasted peppers
  a cup of finely diced celery (1.5 cups) 1 red onion, diced (about 0.25 cup).
  freshly chopped parsley (0.25 cup), if available 2 tablespoons of pumpkin seeds a tablespoon of sunflower seeds 2 teaspoons of sesame seeds
  To make the dressing, combine lime juice and 2 tablespoons fresh Tahini in a small bowl.

3 tablespoons of apple cider vinegar 1 teaspoon maple syrup according to taste with salt and freshly ground black pepper Prepare your baking sheet by preheating the oven to 375°F.

Combine the almonds, maple syrup, and tamari in a large mixing bowl until well blended. Using a fork, toss the almonds with sea salt and drizzle the coconut oil over the top.

Create an even layer of almonds on a baking sheet by covering it with aluminum foil.

Stirring and turning the almonds every 15 to 20 minutes, for about 15 to 20 minutes is sufficient.

Add all of the dressing ingredients to a jar and shake vigorously until everything is well combined while the almonds are toasting.

Allow to cool on a plate or in a bowl after the almonds have completed their toasting process.

All of the remaining salad ingredients should be mixed together in a large mixing bowl. Combine the salad ingredients by pouring some dressing over it and mixing thoroughly.

There are eleven individual servings in this recipe.

Garlic and spinach are two of the most nutritious vegetables you can eat!

5-ounce serving of fresh spinach Bacon (chopped) Balsamic Vinegar (two cloves) 2 dashes of vinegar 6 teaspoons extra-virgin olive oil.

Add a dash of cracked black pepper to taste. Take it with a grain of salt

Slowly cook the garlic in oil over a very low heat until it is softened. Cook, stirring constantly, until the garlic is fragrant; make sure not to let it burn.

Fresh spinach should be added to the pan and mixed with the garlic mixture.

Make sure to cook the fresh spinach for just a few minutes until it begins to wilt. Season with salt and pepper to taste, then serve in a bowl with a few dashes of balsamic vinegar.

This recipe serves two people.

The rice with turmeric is a traditional dish in India.

1 cup brown rice (rinsed thoroughly) 1.75 quarts of chicken broth 1, diced onion, 8 ounces of finely chopped coriander, 1 teaspoon of ground turmeric 3 teaspoons finely chopped garlic The following amounts are in teaspoons: 1 teaspoon paprika

1 teaspoon of cumin powder 0.5 teaspoon of freshly ground black pepper 0.5 teaspoon of sea salt

To make the oil, heat it up in a small saucepan over a medium heat. Cook the onion, stirring frequently, for approximately 8 minutes.

Cook for another 60 seconds after combining the garlic and onion. a b

Then, while stirring constantly, add the broth, rice, cumin, turmeric, pepper, salt, and paprika to the pan and combine everything together well. Start by bringing the water to a boil on the stovetop on medium high heat.

Soon after the rice begins to boil, lower the heat to low and let it simmer in the covered saucepan for 15 minutes or so. Add another 40 minutes to the rice's cooking time. Then turn off the heat, but keep the lid on so that the rice can continue to steam for about 10 minutes.

Using a fork, gently stir in the brown rice and cilantro until well combined.

It serves 6 people.

Frites de pommes de terre dulces

6 teaspoons coconut oil, melted Sweet Potato - 1 teaspoon Turmeric powder - 1 teaspoon 0.5 tsp sea salt (as needed) with ground cinnamon

Set the oven to 425 degrees Fahrenheit and bake for 30 minutes.

In a medium-sized mixing bowl, combine the potato strips with the coconut oil and spices and toss well.

Make sure all of the potatoes are well coated.

Fries should be baked in a single layer on a baking sheet for about 8 to 10 minutes, then the sweet potatoes should be flipped and baked for another 10 minutes more.

Afterwards, relax and enjoy yourself.

1 to 2 servings from this recipe

A papaya salad is a refreshing and healthy dish.

Julienned green papaya (three cups) 0.5 cup finely sliced sweet onion (optional). 5. cup of bean sprouts sugar cane (finely diced) - 2 teaspoons 0.25 cup fresh lime juice

2 teaspoons of fish sauce

freshly grated lime zest (0.225 teaspoon) peppercorns, freshly ground

Hot or Hawaiian chiles, chopped fresh from the garden

Combine the fish sauce, lime juice, sugar, chilies, and zest in a large mixing bowl until well combined and well blended.

In a medium-sized mixing bowl, blend the papaya, bean sprouts, and onion until well incorporated. Before serving, season with freshly ground pepper to taste.

It serves 6 people.

Dishes that are vegetarian.

Quinoa Salad with Turmeric

Potatoes - 7 small (yellow) Quinoa - 1/4 cup Chickpeas - 1 15-ounce can 2 tablespoons of turmeric 1 teaspoon of paprika

2 leaves of kale

avocado + 1 tablespoon coconut oil = 0.5 teaspoons olive oil = 1 tablespoon When required, season with pepper and salt

Temperature: 350 degrees Fahrenheit (fan forced oven).

Make strips out of the yellow potatoes and put them out on a baking pan.

In a small bowl, combine the coconut oil and 1 teaspoon turmeric and drizzle over the potatoes, softly coating them. Depending on your preference, season with pepper and salt.

While you drain and rinse the chickpeas, bake the potatoes for a few minutes. In a large mixing basin, combine the chickpeas with 1 teaspoon paprika and stir well. The chickpeas should be placed on a baking sheet after the potatoes are removed from the oven.

To soften the potatoes, bake the chickpeas and potatoes together for approximately 25 minutes at 350°F.

In a small saucepan, bring the quinoa to a boil. Pepper, salt, and 1 teaspoon of turmeric should be added after the meat has been cooked. Allow to cool after mixing well.

Olive oil should be rubbed into the leaves of the kale after it has been cleaned. Make four separate bowls out of the lettuce leaves. Cut the avocado into thin slices and divide it among the four dishes evenly.

Toss the quinoa with the roast potatoes and chickpeas before plating.

This recipe serves four people.

Lemon Soy Barley Shell (also known as Lemon Soy Barley Shell)

boiling pearl barley (also known as pearl barley or pearl barley): 2 cups 1 cup Organic Edam (peeled) - 0.75 cup

Tofu - Organic Tofu - 2.25 cups (either firm or extra firm) Baked Ripe Avocado - 1 large block, peeled, seeded, cut in half and thinly sliced.

Low Sodium Soy Sauce - 6 tablespoons (for the Lemon Tahini Dressing). 3 tablespoons of toasted sesame seed oil 1.5 tablespoons of dried oregano

Citrus Juice - 0.5 teaspoon coarsely grated lemon

5. a lemon's worth of juice

In a medium saucepan, bring barley and water to a boil.

Once the water has come to a boil, turn the heat down to low and let the barley to simmer for 40 to 50 minutes, depending on how big your pot is. When all of the liquid has been absorbed, the process is considered complete.

Removing the barley from the stove and allowing it to cool will help it absorb some of the flavors.

Using a large mixing bowl, thoroughly blend the sesame oil, oregano, soy sauce, lemon zest, and lemon juice until well incorporated.

In a large mixing basin, combine the cooled barley and the soy mixture, stirring to coat the grain evenly.

Gently fold in the Edam and arugula into the barley mixture until everything is evenly distributed. 14-inch pieces of tofu should be cut.

Divide the barley mixture into four dishes and top with avocado slices and tofu before serving. *

This recipe serves four people.

Salad Sandwiches with Avocado & Egg

1. Avocado, ripe and pitted,.5 teaspoon avocado oil

Organic Hard-Boiled Eggs - 3 oz. each 1 teaspoon freshly squeezed lemon juice

1 celery stalk, coarsely chopped (0.25″ cup total). 3 tablespoons finely minced fresh chives 0.25 teaspoon salt

0.125 tablespoons freshly ground black pepper.

4 pieces of whole wheat sandwich bread 2 leaves of lettuce

Scrape half an avocado into a medium-sized mixing basin and mix with the lemon juice and avocado oil until well combined. Blend until the mixture is practically smooth (around 30 seconds).

In a separate bowl, combine the avocado mixture with the celery, pepper, salt, eggs, and chives, mixing well.

Make two sandwiches by spreading the mixture on two pieces of bread and sandwiching them together with a lettuce leaf and another slice of toast..

This recipe serves two people.

Sweet Potatoes With Stuffing

To make this dish, you will need: 1 big sweet potato 1 cup dried black beans 1 cup canned black beans 1 cup washed and drained Hummus 1.25 cups kale 1.75 cups chopped water 2 tbsp

Poke many holes in the sweet potato with a fork, then place it in the microwave on high for 7 to 10 minutes.

Remove the kale from the water and set it aside to dry. Medium heat and a lid are required to cook the kale. The kale has to be stirred many times so that it becomes wilt.

If the pot is dry, add the beans and 1 to 2 tablespoons water.

Cover the pan and continue to cook the beans and kale until the mixture is heated, approximately 1 to 2 minutes more, stirring often.

Fill the sweet potato with the beans and kale after slicing it in half lengthwise. Serve immediately.

Filling: In a small bowl, combine the hummus and 2 tablespoons of water until desired consistency is reached, then pour over the filled potato to serve.

1 serving (approximately):

Carrots and onions in oil

4 cups of fresh broccoli florets The following ingredients: fresh ginger - 0.25 cup, chopped garlic - 12 cloves, chopped green onions - 1 bunch, cut into slices crushed water chestnuts (one cup) 1 cup chopped mushrooms 1 cup snow peas 1 cup red peppers 1 sliced sesame oil 1 tablespoon sesame seeds If you want to offer brown rice, you may do so.

2 tablespoons reduced sodium soy sauce 1 cup reduced sodium soy sauce 1 cup reduced sodium soy sauce Sesame oil (0.25) cup Cornstarch (one tablespoon)

On a medium-high heat, bring the sesame oil to a boil.

Cook for 20 to 25 minutes, stirring regularly to prevent scorching, after which add the peppers, water chestnuts, snow peas, mushrooms, onion, garlic, broccoli, and ginger to the oil.

In a mason jar, add the first three ingredients and shake vigorously until well-combined (about 30 seconds). As the sauce simmer, it will thicken.

Cook for another 3 to 5 minutes until the veggies are cooked but not too tender and all of the liquid has drained from the pan before adding the stir-fry sauce. Stir often to ensure that the sauce coats all of the veggies properly before serving.

You may eat the fried meal on its own or with brown rice if you choose.

It serves 6 people.

Chapter Seven

Chili in a Crock-Pot

Tomatoes - 3 cups chopped Kidney beans - 3 cups drained and rinsed water.5 cup mushrooms 8 ounces sliced onion 1 diced green peppers 1 chopped garlic cloves 2 minced garlic cloves 2 minced minced garlic cloves 2 minced minced garlic cloves

Corn kernels, either fresh or frozen (not canned) Zucchini: 1 cup - 1 diced chili powder: 1 teaspoon - 6 tablespoons 2-tablespoons of cumin 1/2 tsp cayenne pepper (or to taste) oregano

In a saucepan, add all of the ingredients and stir by hand until everything is well blended. 7 hours on low heat with the lid on

This recipe serves four people.

The Soup of the Month is Butternut Squash

A couple of butternut squashes, peeled and sliced one apple, peeled and chopped a cup of vegetable stock

0.5 cup finely chopped onion

0.55 liters (0.5 cup) heavy whipping cream 1-tablespoon of salt

Peppercorns, 0.125 teaspoon cayenne pepper

Spray the pan with nonstick spray and then add all of the ingredients, except the heavy cream, to the pan and combine. Make a well in the middle of the table and add everything.

Turn up the heat to high and cook for 4-5 hours on the stove top.

Place half of the pumpkin soup in a blender and mix until smooth and free of lumps. Repeat with the remaining pumpkin soup until all of the pumpkin soup has been blended.

Remove half of the pumpkin mixture and puree it again, then pour the soup into a large mixing bowl and serve immediately.

Put everything back into the slow cooker saucepan and whisk in the heavy cream with a hand mixer until everything is smooth.

Replace the cover of the slow cooker and let the soup to simmer for a few more minutes, until it is well cooked and well-combined (around 15 minutes).

It serves 6 people.

Pumpkin Penne with a Crispy Crumby Crumby Crumby Crumby Crumby Crumby

Squash:\sDelicata squash (two medium, washed and rinsed). 2 tablespoons sea salt (as required) in olive oil.

when you need it, freshly ground black pepper

Pesto made from walnuts:

1.25 cups chopped fresh parsley 1.25 cups toasted walnut halves 3 cloves of garlic

6 big leaves of sage. Salted Toasted Walnut Oil (as required) -.5 cup

when you need it, freshly ground black pepper

Ingredients: Whole Wheat Penne noodles, uncooked Parmesan cheese, grated Extra Virgin Olive Oil, and fresh sage leaves for frying (optional).

Prepare your baking pan by preheating the oven to 425°F.

Placing a silicone pad on a tray and setting it away until you are ready to use it Preparing the noodles requires boiling salted water.

Squash should be cut in half lengthwise once the ends are removed. Using a spoon, scrape the seeds out of the pumpkin.

Make 12″ crescent-shaped slices out of each squash half and arrange them on a baking sheet coated with parchment paper.

Season the pumpkin with pepper and salt after drizzling it with olive oil. To prevent them from touching one other, spread them evenly in the pan.

After roasting the squash in the oven for 10 to 15 minutes, take the squash from the oven and flip it over. The squash should be tender after 10 to 12 minutes of frying.

Then, while the squash is roasting, use a food processor to finely chop together the walnuts, parsley, garlic, and sage leaves. Continue to pulse until the mixture is virtually smooth, then add the walnut oil. Place the pesto in a large mixing bowl and season with pepper and sea salt to taste.

A small plate should be covered with paper towels, and a tiny quantity of olive oil should be heated over medium-high heat.

Season with salt and pepper and fry a few sage leaves at a time until crisp, then move to the dish with the cover. Place the mixture in a small bowl and season gently with salt and pepper.

Fill a large saucepan halfway with boiling water and cook the noodles until they're tender. Set aside 8 ounces of the water in which the noodles were cooked, and then drain the noodles to remove any residual water. A little amount of olive oil should be drizzled over the spaghetti and mixed thoroughly. In a large mixing bowl, combine the pasta, grated parmesan cheese, and pesto. Gently toss the noodles in the sauce until they are equally covered. Pour in a little amount of the pasta water that was set aside to make the sauce creamier, if required.

The noodles should be served with the pumpkin chunks on top and a garnish of crispy sage leaves.

4-6 people may be fed using this recipe.

Cooked curry potatoes with an egg on top

To make this dish, you'll need: 2 russet potatoes, 15 ounce can of tomato sauce, 4 big organic eggs, 1 inch of fresh ginger, 3 teaspoons of garlic, 2 teaspoons of curry powder, 2 tablespoons of olive oil, 2 cloves of garlic, 2 teaspoons of curry powder. Chop up 0.5 bunch of fresh cilantro.

Remove the potatoes from the water and cut them into cubes about 3 inches in diameter. Cover the potatoes with water in a big saucepan and set aside.

Using a tight-fitting cover, bring the water to a boil on a high heat. The potatoes should be cooked until they are readily punctured with a fork, then drained well.

Peel the ginger with a vegetable peeler and shred around 1″ of ginger with a tiny perforated grater before chopping the garlic and adding it to the dish.

Heat 1 to 2 tablespoons olive oil in a large pan over medium/low heat for 1 to 2 minutes, then add the curry and cook for another minute or two, until the curry is fragrant.

Slowly bring the heat up to a medium-high setting and gently pour in the sauce. Make sure to stir constantly so that the sauce does not burn. Afterwards, taste it and adjust the seasonings as needed.

The potatoes should be coated evenly in the pan.

4 little dips should be formed in the potato mixture, and 1 egg should be placed in each one. Remove from the heat and continue to cook for 6 to 10 minutes, stirring occasionally, until the eggs are done to your preference.

Fresh coriander should be added at the end.

This recipe serves four people.

Chapter Eight

Salmon Tartine with Smoked Salmon

Clarified butter - 2 tablespoons for making potato tartine

1 big russet potato - 1 large russet potato that has been peeled and shredded As required, season with black pepper and salt.

Toppings:

4 ounces of soft goat cheese at room temperature is plenty. 1.5% of the total weight of the ingredients.

1 cup coarsely sliced red onion, 2 teaspoons 1 cup capers (drained), 2 teaspoons

1 hard-boiled egg, finely chopped 1 garlic clove, chopped 1 hard-boiled egg, finely chopped 1 smoked salmon, thinly sliced half-lemon zest

Garnishing with finely chopped chives

Combine the garlic, lemon zest, and goat cheese in a large mixing bowl until well combined. Toss in the chives and season with salt and black pepper before setting aside.

Hard-boiled eggs and red onion should be lightly salted.

Gradually shred the potato into a large mixing bowl by hand, using the big-hole grater. Remove extra moisture from the potato by squeezing it over a sink or basin.

Make liberal use of pepper and salt while seasoning the potatoes. Over medium-high heat, melt the ghee in a nonstick skillet.

Then, after the butter has been cooked, form the grated potatoes into a huge circular pattern in the pan using a spatula.

The potatoes should be returned to the heated pan with the help of a spatula. Cook the potatoes, covered, for approximately 8 minutes, or until they are golden.

Allow for about 8 minutes of browning on the opposite side after gently turning the pan around.

As soon as the potatoes are crispy and golden brown, take them from the pan and set them aside to rest on a cooling rack until they are at room temperature.

Then, on top of the potato cake, spread the goat cheese.

To assemble, layer the smoked salmon on top of the cheese mixture and garnish with the hard-boiled egg, capers, and red onion, if desired.

Slice the potatoes into wedges and garnish with chives, if using.

1 to 2 servings from this recipe

Shrimp and Avocado Salad (with Quinoa)

The following ingredients are needed to make Crispy Kale: 2 tablespoons olive oil 1 bunch kale, coarsely shredded freshly ground pepper and salt to taste

Quinoa: 2 teaspoons olive oil, 1.25 cups quinoa, 2 cups chicken broth, salt, and pepper to taste

Shrimp and Toppings with a Spicy Twist

Deveined and skinned shrimp weighing 1 pound Ripe avacados - 2 (peeled, cored, and sliced) Watermelon Radishes - 2 Thinly sliced 3 tablespoons of extra virgin olive oil a teaspoon of cumin powder, 2 teaspoons of hot sauce 0.75 teaspoon salt and pepper - powdered coriander

To bake, preheat the oven to 400°F. A silicone pad should be used to line a baking sheet.

Olive oil and kale should be combined. Add pepper and salt to taste, if desired, before serving.

Place the kale on a baking sheet so that it does not overlap, and then cook until it becomes crispy. (12-15 minutes) (about The oil should be heated in a medium saucepan over medium-high heat while the kale is roasting in the oven.

Stir regularly while toasting the quinoa in the olive oil for approximately 1 minute in a skillet over medium-high heat.

Simmer the quinoa in the broth for about 15 minutes after carefully pouring it over it in the pot.

Continue to cook the quinoa until there is no more liquid and the quinoa has softened, around 20 minutes. Season the quinoa with a pinch of pepper and salt and leave it aside for the time being,

On a medium-high heat, heat the oil in a saucepan.

Stir together the shrimp, cumin, coriander, and spicy sauce in a medium-sized mixing bowl until well-coated.

Season the shrimp with salt and pepper before cooking them in the pan for 4 to 5 minutes, or until they are cooked through.

Separate the quinoa into four bowls and arrange kale and shrimp on top of each.

Remove from heat and quickly top each bowl with the slices of avocado and watermelon radish.

This recipe serves four people.

Taco Wrapped with Salmon

2 filets of wild salmon

Collard Salad Dressing or Shredded Cabbage - 2 or 3 cups Fresh cilantro - 0.25 cup lettuce - 1 head

1.5 tablespoons of seasoning for grilled fish. 1 lime juice, 1 teaspoon salt, to taste 1 avocado oil

Ingredients for mayonnaise: 1 cup avocado oil - 1 cup organic egg - 1 large lemon juice - 1 teaspoon salt 0.25 teaspoon salt

0.5 teaspoon of Dijon mustard

Avocado sauce (0.5 avocado, pitted): Avocado (0.5 avocado, pitted) 1 cup chopped fresh cilantro 1 cup seeded jalapeno 25 cup water 1 clove garlic 1 teaspoon salt 0.5 teaspoon salt

In order to begin, combine all of the ingredients in a glass jar and mix until smooth using an immersion blender (optional). Allowing for the egg to be carried along with it, bring the blender all the way down to the bottom of the jar and blend at the bottom until the mixture is white and creamy, then gently lift the blender back up to ensure that everything is well blended and completed

To make the avocado sauce, first combine all of the ingredients in a blender with 1/2 cup mayonnaise and mix until completely smooth. If you wish to thin the sauce, add a little water and continue to combine.

Drizzle a little avocado oil over each piece of salmon after topping with the grilled fish seasoning and dabbing gently to ensure that the seasoning adheres properly.

Preheat the grill to medium-high heat and cook the salmon for 5 to 8 minutes, rotating once, until it is opaque throughout. Keep them from drying out by overcooking them. Set aside the salmon after it has cooled down after it has been removed from the grill.

Chop the cilantro and lime juice and combine them in a small dish with the coleslaw. Salt to taste (optional).

Using a paper towel, dry off the lettuce leaves once they have been rinsed. For the taco wraps, use the nicest cup-shaped leaves available.

As soon as the salmon has been allowed to cool, chop it up and lay it in the lettuce wraps, gently covering it with the lettuce mixture.

The tacos should be topped with the avocado sauce.

4-6 people may be fed using this recipe.

Fish and shellfish are Chaudrauf's specialities.

Fillet of salmon (.33 lb) without skin Cod fillets weighing.33 pound each Bone Broth - 1 cup full-fat coconut cream -.5 cup white sweet potato - 1 small, peeled and diced fennel bulb - 1 small, finely chopped carrots - 3 celery ribs, peeled and sliced 3. Thyme, finely chopped - 1.5 tablespoons olive oil, chopped - 3 tablespoons bay leaf, finely chopped - 1 teaspoon fine sea salt, to taste

Stockpot over medium-high heat for approximately 10 minutes while sautéing the celery, carrots, sweet potato, fennel bulb, thyme, and bay leaf in hot olive oil. Toss the ingredients often. Watch carefully so that the veggies do not brown or adhere to the pan; if necessary, add extra oil.

Pour in the broth slowly, stirring constantly, and bring the pot to a boil over medium high heat. Pour in the fish and reduce the heat to medium-low while the fish cooks. 8-10 minutes more cooking time is required after that.

Using a slotted spoon, transfer the fish to a serving platter when the veggies have softened and the fish has been cooked. Remove and discard the bay leaf. Take care to remove any residual bones from the fish before slicing it into smaller pieces.

After the fish pieces have been returned to the pot with the coconut cream, give them a quick stir. Add a little of salt to the soup if you like it.

Just before serving, garnish with fresh thyme.

This recipe serves four people.

The Fajitas del Mar del Mar del Mar del Mar

1.5 pounds fresh shrimp, seeded and peeled Yellow peppers - 1 thinly sliced (optional) 1. one thinly sliced red pepper; 1. one small, thinly sliced red onion; 1. one orange bell pepper; and 1. one tablespoon of extra-virgin olive oil.

0.5 teaspoon ground garlic

0.5 tablespoons of chili powder 1-tablespoon of salt

0.5 teaspoon ground cumin The following amounts are in teaspoons: 1 teaspoon paprika

0.5 teaspoon of lime juice and onion powder

tortillas that have been reheated

450 degrees Fahrenheit should be set in the oven.

Combine the paprika, olive oil, shrimp, onion, pepper, salt, and spices in a large mixing bowl until everything is well combined. Ensure a thorough mixing.

Preparation: Spray a sheet pan with nonstick cooking spray and arrange the ingredients in such a way that none of them overlap the others.

Fry for approximately 8 minutes, then reduce the heat to low and continue to fry for 2 minutes longer to finish cooking the shrimp

When you take out the fajita mixture from the oven, drizzle it with lime juice. Serve in tortillas, garnished with fresh coriander, and enjoy!

This recipe serves four people.

Mediterranean cod is a type of cod that is native to the Mediterranean region.

Scallops (one pound, cut into four servings): Tomatoes (diced) - 1 can (14.5 oz) Tomato sauce kale (about 2 cups, shredded) - 2-cups thinly sliced fennel.

2 cups finely chopped, fresh-picked tomatoes 1 cup of black olives

.5 cup of water

Small onion (sliced thinly) 2 tablespoons extra virgin olive oil

3 large cloves of garlic, peeled and finely minced 2 teaspoons of fresh oregano 0.125 teaspoons of sea salt

0.25 teaspoon ground fennel

0.25 teaspoons freshly ground black pepper 1 teaspoon of orange zest

crushed red pepper flakes (optional)

Decorate with fresh oregano, fennel fronds, olive oil, orange peel, and other herbs and vegetables as a garnish

Using a medium-high flame, heat the oil. Season the fennel, garlic, and onion with pepper and salt after 8 minutes of cooking in the oil. Combine the water, tomatoes, and kale in a large mixing bowl until thoroughly combined. Pour in the milk and stir until everything is well combined. Simmer for 10 to 12 minutes until everything is well combined.

Season with salt, freshly ground pepper, oregano, and olives before adding them to the pan. Orange zest, pepper, fennel seeds, and salt are used to season the fish before cooking it in the oven.

Place the fish in a bowl with the tomato and cabbage mixture and cover with plastic wrap.

Allow the fish to cook through for approximately 10 minutes before turning off the heat. Garnish the mixture with fresh herbs and serve it right away.

This recipe serves four people.

Chapter Nine

Salmon with zucchini and lemon dressing

Seafood: 4 salmon fillets (each weighing 5 ounces) Chop up two heads of garlic (two cloves). 0.5 teaspoon dried dill

2 tablespoons of brown sugar, tightly sealed 0.5 teaspoon dried oregano

a couple of tablespoons of lemon juice (freshly squeezed) parsley (freshly chopped) - 6 teaspoons

1 tablespoon of Dijon mustard 0.25 tsp of dried rosemary 0.25 teaspoon dried thyme

As required, season with freshly ground black pepper and salt

4 pieces of zucchini, chopped 2 tablespoons extra virgin olive oil to taste - season with salt and pepper

Preheat the oven to 400°F and lightly grease a baking pan with cooking spray before beginning.

Then combine the Dijon mustard with the brown sugar, dill and lemon juice, as well as the herbs (thyme, rosemary, garlic, and oregano), and set aside. Set aside after adding pepper and salt.

On a baking sheet, arrange the courgettes in an even layer and season with pepper and salt before sprinkling with olive oil. Arrange the salmon fillets on a baking sheet and brush them with the herb mix.

Preparing the fish in the oven takes 16 to 18 minutes, depending on how flaky the fish is when it is done. Add a sprig of parsley on top and serve!

This recipe serves four people.

meatballs

2.25 lbs. of ground beef

1 teaspoon coriander, pre-measured 5-cloves of garlic, pressed firmly together 1/2 teaspoon ground ginger 1 teaspoon sea salt 1/8 teaspoon lime zest

Heat the oven to 350 degrees Fahrenheit.

Set aside a baking sheet that has been lined with aluminum foil.

Form the mixture into 12 equal-sized balls by combining it all with your hands. 20 to 25 minutes, or until meatballs are slightly pink in the center, should be enough time to bake them.

Sea salt should be sprinkled over the meatballs before serving with a green salad on the side.

This recipe serves four people.

Casserole with Bacon and Cheddar

2.25 lbs. of ground beef

3 cups sweet potato (rolled) 1 cup green onion (roughly chopped) 1 cup

0.5% coconut cream from a 13.5-ounce can of coconut milk Bacon without nitrates - 8 slices, cooked and crumbled 1 teaspoon of table salt

Ingredients: 1 teaspoon nutritional yeast, 2 tablespoons coconut oil

375 degrees Fahrenheit should be set in the oven. You can cook the bacon in any way you want and then set it aside to rest.

The sweet potatoes should be steamed until they are cooked through, but not mushy. In a water bath or in the microwave with a small amount of water, steam them until they are tender.

Using a cast iron skillet, heat the coconut oil until it is completely melted. Once the oil is hot, add the ground beef and 12 teaspoon sea salt and cook until the beef is cooked through. When it has been cooking for a few minutes, add the green onion and 2-1/2 cups of the steamed potatoes to the pot. Cook until the beef is browned and the sweet potatoes are lightly caramelized, about 15 minutes total time

Combine the ground beef mixture with the cooked bacon by crumbling it over the top and stirring until everything is well-incorporated.

Open the can of coconut cream after it has been shaken for about a minute. In a blender, blend half of these ingredients together with the yeast, 14 teaspoon salt, and the remaining sweet potato until smooth. Combine all of the ingredients in a blender until thoroughly combined.

Place the pan in the oven for approximately 5 minutes after pouring the sauce from the blender over the ground beef mix.

Pickles and red onions should be served on the side to complete the meal.

It serves 6 people.

Hummus in Gold

1 can (15 ounces) chickpeas, drained 1 medium lemon (1 medium lemon juice)

Grated Olive Oil - 1.5 tablespoons, 0.5 tablespoons grated Ginger 3 tablespoons of tahini 0.5 teaspoon grated turmeric 0.25 teaspoon ground turmeric Chop up two heads of garlic (two cloves).

0.25 teaspoon fine sea salt

The cayenne pepper is a pinch of it.

All of the ingredients in the ingredient list should be blended until smooth in a blender or food processor. Adjust seasonings as needed after tasting the hummus.

Refrigerate for 3 to 4 days if stored in an airtight container or bag.

Ranch Dressing with Coconut Milk 1 liter of coconut cream (ingredients should be just coconut and water) 2 tablespoons finely chopped shallots

Chopped chives (0.125 cup total)

2.25 tablespoons of apple cider vinegar. 1.5 tablespoons fresh basil, finely minced

chopped dill (2.75% of a teaspoon) 2 tablespoons parsley, finely diced 0.75 teaspoons of fine sea salt Chopped garlic (one clove)

Then, using a spoon, carefully scoop out the coconut cream, leaving the water in its container. 4 tablespoons coconut water should be whisked into the cream.

Add the remaining ingredients from the ingredients list to the mixing bowl and stir until everything is well combined.

Refrigerate for at least 30 minutes before serving to allow the flavors to meld together fully.

Mustard

Apple Cider Vinegar -.25 cup Raw honey - 1 tablespoon Ingredients 0.5 cup freshly ground mustard 0.25 teaspoon fine sea salt 0.25 teaspoon of ground turmeric

Then, in a small mixing bowl, thoroughly combine all of the ingredients. Refrigerator storage is recommended in a tightly closed jar. a spicy condiment

Apple Cider Vinegar -.25 cup Tomato paste - 1 tablespoon Ingredients 1.25 cup of water

25 grams (0.225 tablespoon) of hot pepper paprika 0.5 teaspoon cayenne pepper 0.25 teaspoon fine sea salt

0.125 teaspoons crushed red pepper flakes. 0.125 teaspoons of minced garlic

All of the ingredients listed in the ingredient list should be mixed together thoroughly in a mixing bowl. Refrigerator storage is recommended in a tightly closed jar. Mayonnaise

Egg (Organic) 1 Large Avocado Oil (Eight Ounces)

1.5 tbsp. apple cider vinegar (optional) 1.25 teaspoons Dijon mustard (optional)

0.25 teaspoon fine sea salt

Then blend the mixture in a blender until it is smooth.

While the blender is running, slowly drizzle in the avocado oil through the funnel and continue to blend until the mixture is thick.

Fill an airtight jar with the mayo after it has been thoroughly mixed with the avocado oil. Refrigerate for up to 2 weeks.

The pesto made from dandelion flowers

Dandelion leaves - 2 cups, crushed and loosely packed Dandelion leaves Freshly grated Parmesan cheese and pine nuts equal 0.25 cup; 4 ounces of extra-virgin olive oil.

3 cloves of garlic, crushed 1 tablespoon lemon juice 0.5 teaspoon table salt

1 tablespoon of lemon zest 1 teaspoon of turmeric powder

Blend all of the ingredients from the ingredients list, with the exception of the cheese, in a blender until completely smooth.

If the pesto is too thick, thin it out with a small amount of olive oil until it reaches the consistency you desire. Blend in the Parmesan cheese until it is completely smooth and creamy.

You should keep it in the refrigerator for no more than 72 hours in an airtight container.

Drinks and smoothies are popular.

Smoothie with lots of greens in it

Frozen banana (sliced): 1 banana 7 1/2 cups fresh kale 8 oz unsweetened almond milk .25 teaspoon turmeric "and sliced after they've been peeled

0.25 oz. grated ginger "0.5 teaspoon of Chia seeds, peeled and sliced

0.25 teaspoon freshly ground cinnamon 0.5 teaspoon ground flaxseed

Using a blender, combine all of the ingredients and process until smooth. Pour the mixture into your glass once it has been thoroughly mixed and liquefied. Fruit Smoothie with Cherries and Bananas

2 ripe bananas, 2 baby spinach, 1 cup coconut water, 0.75 cup ginger, 1 teaspoon freshly grated turmeric powder, 1 teaspoon freshly grated turmeric powder, 1 teaspoon freshly grated turmeric powder, 1 teaspoon freshly grated turmeric powder

75 grams of pre-soaked chia seeds 0.25 teaspoon ground cinnamon

Put everything in a blender and pulse until it's smooth.

Fruit Smoothie with Cherries and Mango

sweet cherries - 1 cup frozen sweet cherries 1 cup frozen mango (optional).

.5 cup of water 1.75 cup of water

Separate the cherries and the mangoes and set them aside to thaw while you prepare the other ingredients. In a blender, combine the cherries with 4 ounces of water and puree.

In order to dilute the mixture, you can add an additional 14 cup of water before pouring it into a glass.

Using a clean blender, puree the mango with the remaining water until it is smooth. Blend until smooth, adding more water if necessary to achieve a smooth consistency.

Pour into a glass on top of the cherry layer and stir well to incorporate.

Smoothie with blueberries

1 cup of almond milk Frozen bananas (one) 1 cup frozen blueberries (optional). 2 handfuls of spinach 0.25 teaspoon cinnamon 1 tablespoon almond butter Peppercorns, 0.125 teaspoon cayenne pepper

In a blender, combine all of the ingredients and blend until well combined. Fill mugs with the mixture once it has been blended well.

Golden milk is a type of milk that has a golden color to it.

1.5 cups of light coconut milk nut milk (unsweetened) – 1.5 cups 0.25 tsp. ground ginger powder

0.5 tablespoons of turmeric powder 0.25 teaspoon ground cinnamon 1 tablespoon of coconut oil

You can use any sweetener of your choice, for example, B. coconut blossom sugar, maple syrup, and so on.

In a small saucepan, whisk together the ingredients and bring to a boil over medium-high heat. Continue to beat the milk frequently until it is warm to the touch but not hot to the touch.

Adjust any of the ingredients if they are not quite right after you turn off the heat.

Remove the cinnamon stick from the dish and serve right away!

This recipe serves two people.

Cocoa infused with turmeric

Ingredients: 1 cup unsweetened almond milk, 1.5 tablespoons unsweetened cocoa powder 2 tablespoons of coconut oil

2 teaspoons of honey

1 teaspoon of ground turmeric The cayenne pepper is a pinch of it.

one or two grinds of freshly ground black pepper

Using a small saucepan, heat the milk while adding the cocoa, coconut oil, and turmeric until it is steaming hot. Bring the mixture to a boil while whisking it.

Turn off the heat and stir in the pepper and cayenne pepper until the pepper is well combined. Allow for a 2-minute resting period before serving the dish. Smoothie made with beetroot and cherry

Cut two small beetroots into quarters that are ready to eat. Almond Milk with Vanilla Extract - 10 oz. The following amounts are for one banana: 0.5 cup, 0.5 cup of frozen pitted cherries, and 1 tablespoon of frozen almonds.

In a blender, combine all of the ingredients. It is ready to serve once the ingredients have been thoroughly mixed and liquefied. Smoothie with Pineapple

Approximately 1.5 cups pineapple chunks (frozen) Orange - 1 peeled orange, 1 cup coconut water

Finely chopped fresh ginger (about 1 tablespoon) 1.25 teaspoons of ground turmeric

0.25 tsp. freshly ground black pepper To make 0.75 teaspoon of chia seeds

In a blender, combine all of the ingredients. Then it's ready to be served after it's been smoothed out. Smoothie with Greek yogurt

Unsweetened Almond Milk - 1 cup Baby Spinach -.25 cup Plain Greek Yogurt -.5 cup Blueberries -.25 cup (fresh or frozen) Unsweetened Almond Milk - 1 cup 1-tablespoon almond butter Ice cubes (three or four)

Put everything in a blender and blend it until smooth. Then it's ready to be served after it's been smoothed out. Shake with cocoa

1 cup of coconut cream

3 tablespoons of cocoa powder strawberries (frozen) - 1.25 cup .5 cup banana and filtered water Honey (1 tablespoon) - 1 honey jar .75 cup of baby spinach

Place everything in a blender and mix well. Pour into mugs once the mixture has been liquefied and thoroughly mixed. Serve as soon as possible after preparing it.